'If only this book was available a ~~~~ ago when I worked in mainstream schools with children on the spectrum. Informative and easy to understand for young children without any jargon. Great for helping young children understand a topic not often talked about positively in mainstream schools and for helping them understand why their friend/ classmate may behave differently. Long overdue.'

– Gill D. Ansell, author of *Working with Asperger Syndrome in the Classroom*

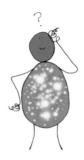

Is It OK to Ask Questions about Autism?

Abi Rawlins

"Ten Tips for Teachers" by Catherine Frizzell
Illustrated by Abi Rawlins
Foreword by Michael Barton

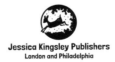

Jessica Kingsley Publishers
London and Philadelphia

First published in 2017
by Jessica Kingsley Publishers
73 Collier Street
London N1 9BE, UK
and
400 Market Street, Suite 400
Philadelphia, PA 19106, USA

www.jkp.com

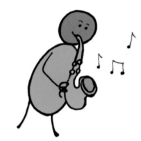

Library of Congress Cataloging in Publication Data
A CIP catalog record for this book is available from the Library of Congress

British Library Cataloguing in Publication Data
A CIP catalogue record for this book is available from the British Library

ISBN 978 1 78592 170 4
eISBN 978 1 78450 439 7

Printed and bound in China

Dedicated to Chris Rawlins and Rob Frizzell

With special thanks to all the people from the autism community who shared their views and experiences so the rest of us may learn

Foreword

I originally met Abi and Catherine at the Autism Show in London on their quest to produce a video explaining what autism is like for a variety of children, from those of primary-school age to me as a young adult. Naturally, I was keen to get on board to give my insight into the world of autism; however, what struck me most was their level of fascination and passion towards the subject of autism, which rivals that of some autistic people who devote themselves to a particular topic!

They're certainly not taking on an easy task. Defining how autism affects a person can be extremely complicated, as autism itself is a very broad subject – it covers every aspect of a person's life. While this means that some people struggle to understand it, it's often the case that simple steps can be taken to reduce many of the anxieties and problems that autistic people face. Sometimes it's just a question of being open-minded and trying to understand things from an autistic person's point of view. Even if something they say or do appears to make no sense, they will almost always have a perfectly logical explanation as an answer.

Many professionals studying the subject research it in a very clinical manner, studying autistic people's behaviours and contemplating what the causes behind them may be. While this research is undoubtedly valuable, I think it's equally important to take the authors' approach and find out about autism from autistic people themselves (there's an expression, 'straight from the horse's mouth', which means exactly that). People often do not appreciate the fact that autism comes as a wide spectrum. The autism community has a saying – 'Once you've met one person with autism, you've met one person with autism'. This emphasises the point that two people can be very different, despite having the same diagnosis.

This book targets people interested in autism and also explains autism in a very clear and understandable manner. It will not only be a useful resource for children, who are often keen to learn about new topics, but it should also enlighten adults about the ways of explaining autism to others. While this book could have been very short (i.e. Is it OK to ask questions? First and only page: Yes), Abi and Catherine have taken the hands-on approach of asking primary-school aged children what questions they would ask about autism and then answering them. This simple yet effective approach is exactly what is needed to educate people on what they need to know about autism.

Michael Barton
author and illustrator of
It's Raining Cats and Dogs and
A Different Kettle of Fish

Introduction

Dear Parents, Schools, Teachers and Allies,

Autism is more common than a lot of people think. There are currently about 700,000 autistic[1] people in the United Kingdom. Being aware of autism and how it can affect people at school or in the workplace will help us make the world a more autism-friendly place.

All the questions in this book were asked by primary-school students. They told us they want to learn about autism so they can be more considerate and understanding of their peers. Their questions are important and merit further exploration. We might not have all the answers yet but we do know enough to educate and empower ourselves with the basics.

As a society we often shy away from talking openly about autism. Some people have told us they are worried they might say the wrong thing, so they end up saying nothing at all. We invite you to use this book as a tool to encourage open and sensitive conversations. On each page you will find digestible information and thoughtful illustrations to help you facilitate discussions about autism within a positive framework.

One of the best ways to learn about autism is to listen to the experiences and views of autistic people. All the answers in this book have been written in collaboration with autistic people and their families. Without their insight this book would not have been possible.

When you ask questions about autism, each autistic person may have a different answer. Think of the answers in this book as a starting point for your own discussions.

Talk about the different ways you could approach each question and encourage young readers to be mindful of other people's feelings and perspectives.

Autism awareness is good for everyone. *Feeling accepted by* others is important, but *being accepting of* others is just as important. We believe everyone should play an active role in creating an environment that acknowledges and values difference. We invite you to create safe and facilitating spaces to share this book and nurture an ethos of collaborative responsibility.

Note

1 We use the term 'autistic' throughout this book because individuals on the spectrum have told us they prefer to be called 'an autistic person', rather than 'a person who has autism'. One reason for this is that you can't separate a person from the way their brain works, it's an intrinsic part of who they are. Saying that a person 'has autism' suggests that autism is something separate that a person can 'have', rather than something they 'are'. When you 'have' something, it implies less permanence and more potential for things such as cures. Many people are proud of their autistic perspectives and they feel that 'being autistic' is not a negative thing, nor does it stop them from having many other qualities and attributes.

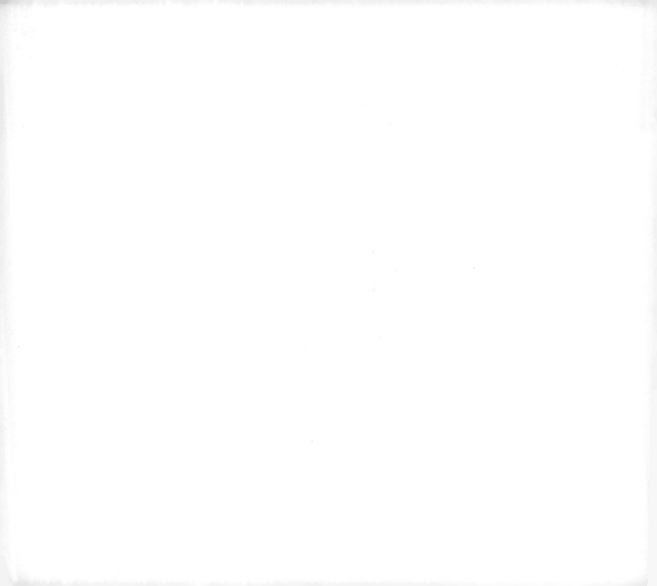

What Is Autism?

Dear Parents. Schools. Teachers and Allies.

In this chapter we will look at some questions and answers that introduce us to the world of autism. Throughout this book we consider the common characteristics of autism. However, it's important to remember that no two individuals are exactly the same. The word autism means different things to different people. As one young person told us, 'We all have different abilities, we all have different needs.'

You can use this book to facilitate discussions and support others to acknowledge and embrace difference. We invite you to share the questions and answers in this book with your family, friends, children and students.

We believe that learning about each other helps us to be more considerate.

Many parents and families work tirelessly to get the right support for their children, under very difficult circumstances. An autistic adult told us, 'Autism can be hard.' However, he also highlighted the positive aspects of autism. There are many autistic adults who are proud of their autism and the unique way they see the world. The following chapters highlight the voices of autistic people who have shared their experiences and differences so that the rest of us may learn.

1. "What is autism?"

Some people are autistic. Autism changes the
way a person thinks and communicates. If you are
autistic, it just means your brain works differently to
someone who isn't autistic. Thinking differently can
help you see the world in new and interesting ways.
Autism can make it harder to understand what other
people are thinking and feeling. If you are autistic
you might feel more sensitive (and sometimes less
sensitive) to everyday sounds, smells, lights and
textures. If your friend is autistic, they might learn or
behave differently to you and that's OK.

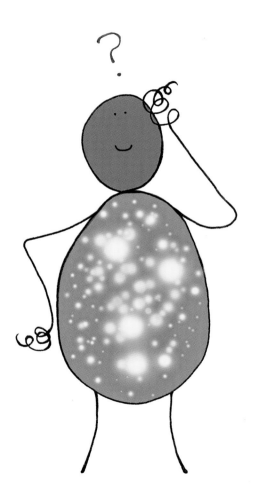

2. "When was autism discovered?"

In 1938, an Austrian doctor called Hans Asperger discovered autism. In 1943, an American doctor wrote a famous report about autism. Both doctors noticed some of their patients behaving in a way they had never seen before. They called the behaviour 'autism'. Our ideas about autism have changed a lot since 1943 and there are still many things to discover about it.

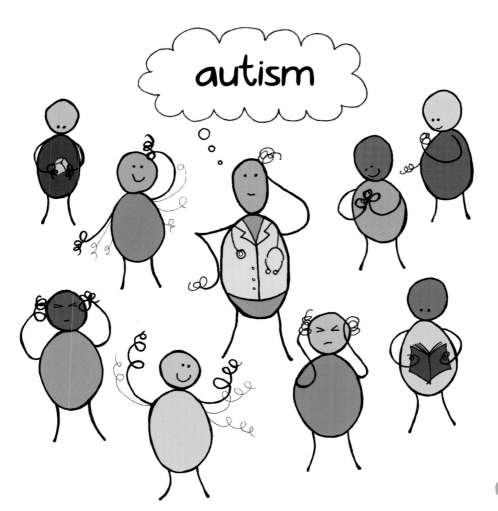

17

3. "How many autistic people are there?"

In the United Kingdom there are more than half a million autistic people. That's one person out of every one hundred people, possibly even more. We don't know how many autistic people there are in the whole world because some countries don't have a record yet. However, we do know that autism is more common than a lot of people think.

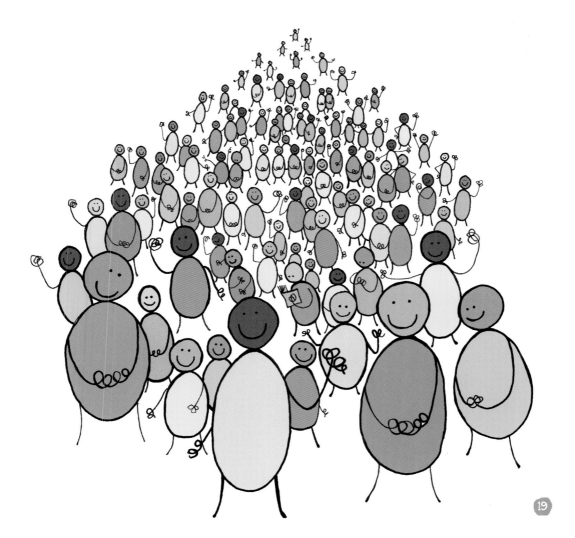

4. "What causes autism?"

We don't know exactly what causes autism. Doctors and scientists have been studying autism for many years and they are still trying to find the cause. There could be more than one thing that causes autism. If you become a scientist or doctor you might discover an answer to this question. Remember, you don't need to know what causes autism in order to be good friends with someone who is autistic.

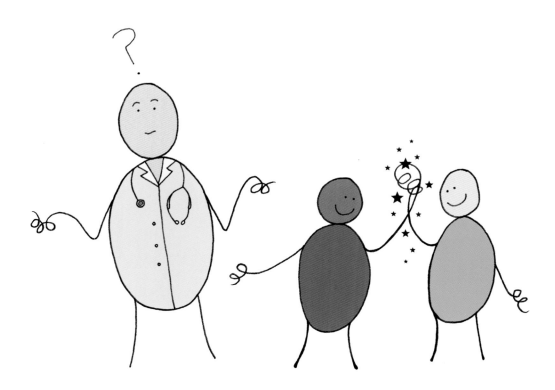

5. "Are there different types of autism?"

Yes, there are lots of different types of autism because there are lots of different types of people. We all have different interests, ideas and strengths. We call autism a 'spectrum' condition, because it affects everyone differently. One autistic person might need more help and support than another autistic person. Autism means different things to different people.

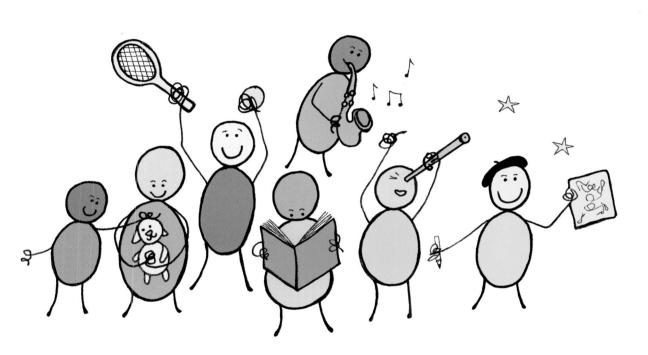

6. "If all autistic people have the same condition, then how does it affect them differently?"

Imagine giving all your friends the same pencils and asking them to draw a picture. It's very unlikely that they would all draw the same picture, even though they used exactly the same pencils. This is because we are all different. Everybody has their own personality and interests, so autism will affect every person differently.

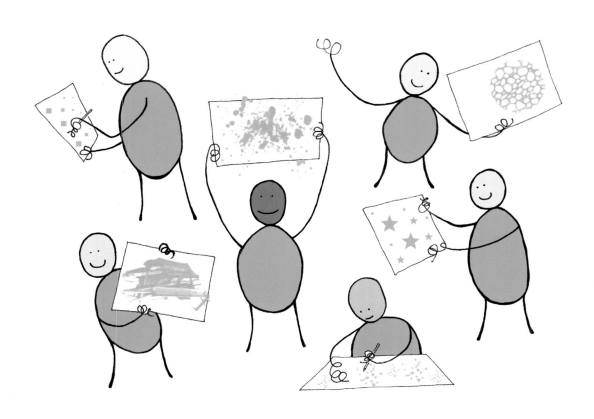

7. "Why is autism called autism?"

The word *autism* comes from the Greek word *autos,* which means 'self'. A long time ago, doctors chose the word *autos* because they thought autistic people were only interested in them*selves*. Now we know that this is completely untrue. Autistic people are very interested in all kinds of different things.

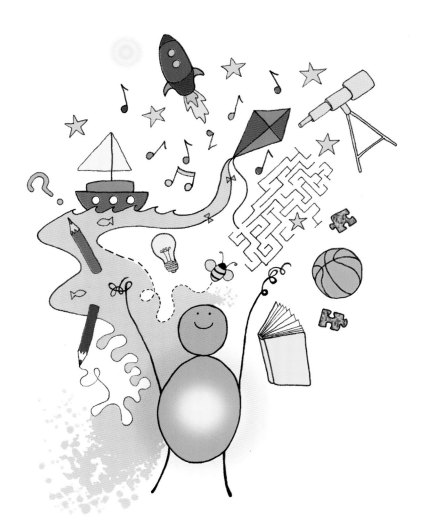

Let's Learn about Autism

Dear Parents, Schools, Teachers and Allies,

In this chapter we will look at some questions and answers to help us understand why autism awareness is so important and the reasons people might not know enough about it. We invite you to consider the individual roles we can play in supporting our society to talk more openly about autism.

A young person told us that some people still don't know much about autism because they haven't spent enough time with autistic people. He also said, 'There aren't really enough things to help them learn about it. There are lots of books but they can be confusing and most of them are aimed at the actual person with autism.'

We have made the questions and answers in this book as digestible as possible and we invite you to bring them to life at home, in the classroom and anywhere you can create a safe and supportive platform for open and sensitive discussion.

A Parent's Perspective...

Whose responsibility is it to ensure that autism is better understood and accepted? A mother who has autistic children and is also autistic herself suggests that the onus of acceptance is currently placed unfairly on the shoulders of those who wish to be accepted. We support her in asking, 'Can the rest of society take more ownership of this responsibility?'

8. "Why is it important to learn about autism?"

Learning about autism is important because it helps us to be more aware and more considerate. Sometimes autistic people are left out because their behaviour is misunderstood by others. It's important to teach ourselves about autism so that we can be more understanding and respectful. If more people learn about autism then the world will be a more autism-friendly place. Many autistic people have unique experiences and ideas to share, so living in an autism-friendly world is good for everyone.

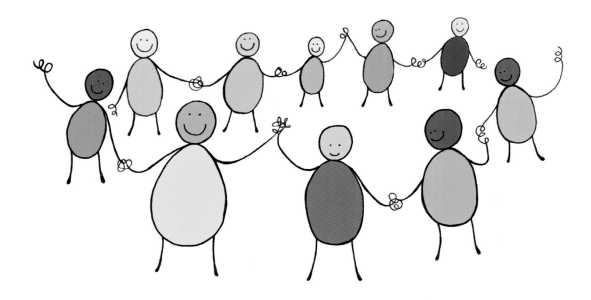

9. "Why don't many people know about autism?"

Some people don't know about autism because nobody in their family is autistic. Many people don't know how to start a conversation about autism. It's hard to learn about autism if you don't talk about it. Some people ignore autism because they are too nervous to ask questions. Other people think they already know the answers. A good way to learn about autism is to make friends with someone who is autistic.

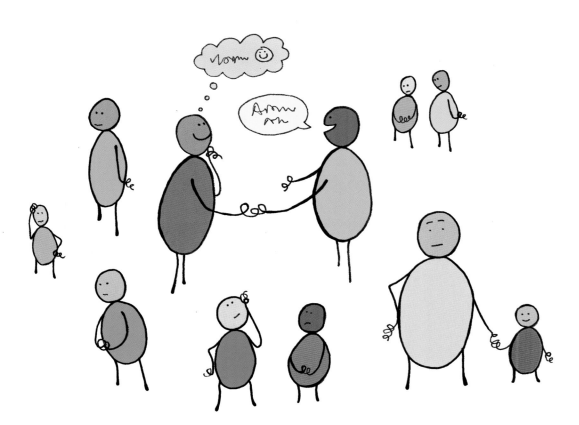

10. "Are there more autistic boys or autistic girls?"

Records show that there are lots more autistic boys than autistic girls. However, there might be more autistic girls than we realise. Sometimes autistic girls don't get the right support because other people don't realise they are autistic. Doctors, parents and teachers could be noticing autism in boys more easily. It's important that everybody gets the support they need.

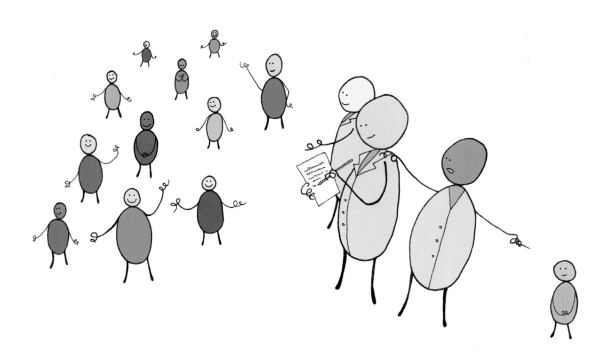

11. "Do autistic people need to be treated differently?"

We all need to be treated differently sometimes. Being treated differently can be a good thing. When it's your birthday you are treated differently and people give you presents. If you are autistic you might get extra help at school. If your friend is autistic and they don't like playing in a crowded place, you could try finding a different place to play. However, if you treat someone differently to make them feel sad or alone, that's not OK.

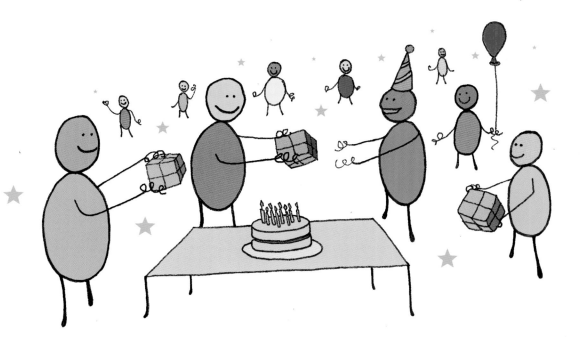

12. "What things are good about autism?"

If you are autistic, it changes the way you see and experience the world. Some people are very proud to be autistic because it gives them useful skills like noticing small details that other people miss. If you are autistic, you might have an interesting hobby that you can stay focused on for hours. Being very focused on a particular subject can help you become a real expert. All autistic people have different personalities, interests and strengths.

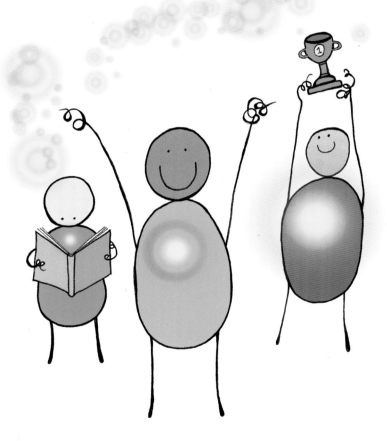

13. "How does autism affect talking?"

Autism affects everybody differently. Some autistic people can speak incredibly well and others cannot speak at all. There are lots of different ways to say things without words. Some people use pictures to show what they are thinking. Other people learn sign language and use their hands to communicate. Just because somebody can't speak with their mouth, it doesn't mean they have nothing to say.

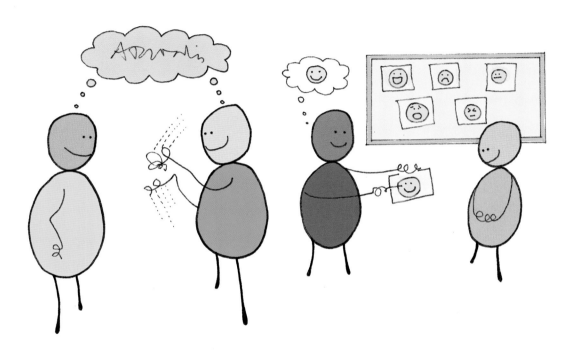

14. "Is there a school for autistic people?"

Yes, your school! There are schools especially for autistic students but all schools should be autism-friendly. Sometimes autistic students need extra support so they go to schools where the teachers know a lot about autism. However, most autistic students go to the same schools as everybody else. How autism-friendly is your school?

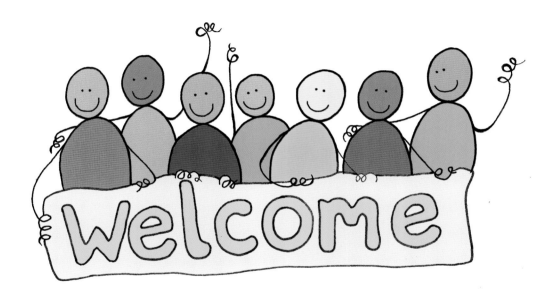

How Can I Be a Good Friend?

Dear Parents. Schools. Teachers and Allies.

In this chapter we consider the questions primary-school students have asked us about playing games, making friends and growing up. We invite you to investigate the information in this chapter and support young readers to consider what social activities and friendship mean to them.

When we asked autistic people and their families how to be a good friend to someone with autism, they frequently prioritised 'learning about autism'. We invite you to reflect on the questions and answers in this chapter and we encourage you to learn about autism by meeting autistic people and listening to their views.

A young person whose brother is autistic said, 'Just talk to them and find out what they're like.' Starting a conversation with somebody who thinks and behaves differently to you can be daunting at first. The answers in this chapter provide ideas to help young readers reflect on common queries about autism in the context of friendship. With the right support and information, neurotypical students can become more aware, accepting and considerate of their autistic peers.

A Parent's Perspective...

Parents told us they would like to highlight the fact that 'playing' can be hard work for individuals on the spectrum. An activity that is of great interest to one person might seem boring to someone else. The questions and answers in the following chapter encourage young readers to find out what their peers enjoy doing for fun. We also introduce readers to the concept of 'literal thinking'.

15. "Is it easy to make friends when you are autistic?"

Some autistic people are good at making friends and others find it more difficult. Everybody is different. Autistic people find it harder to understand what other people are thinking and feeling. Autism makes it difficult to understand facial expressions such as smiles and frowns. If you are autistic, you and your friends might need a bit of help to keep your friendships going. However, you can still have lots of great friendships with many different people.

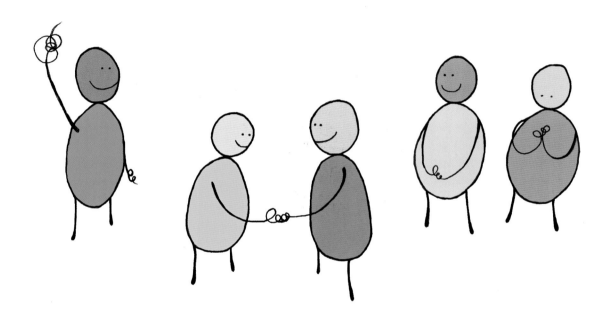

16. "My friend is autistic, how can I help them if they are feeling worried or scared?"

You can try to find out what is upsetting your friend by talking to them. If they are doing things like tapping, flapping or humming, don't try to stop them. If they are feeling anxious because of a busy school corridor you could offer to walk with them to a quieter place. If they are upset about an unexpected change or a friendship problem, you could offer your advice but you might need to ask an adult you trust for extra support and suggestions.

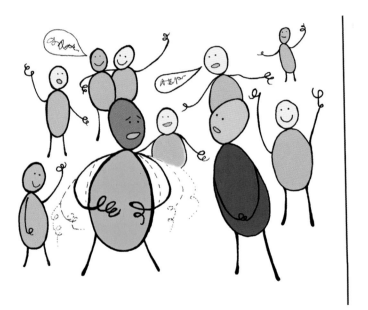
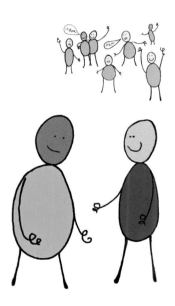

17. "How can you help someone who is autistic to understand games?"

Autism can make it more difficult to join in and play games. Before you begin, find out if your friend wants to play the game. Explain the rules clearly and try speaking one at a time when you are sharing important information. It might be helpful to show your friend how the game works by letting them watch you play it first. Sometimes people might not like playing the same games as you. Have you tried finding out what your friend likes to do for fun?

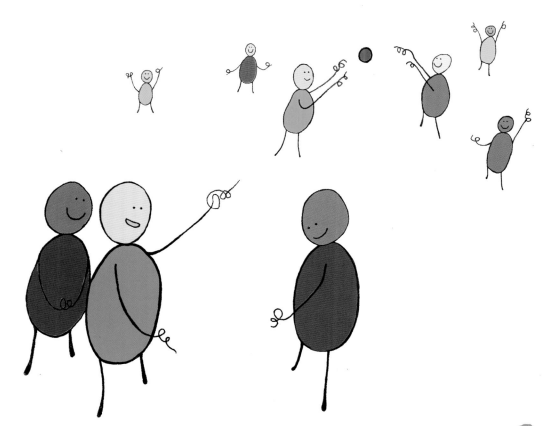

18. "Do autistic people think differently to people who are not autistic?"

Yes, autism changes the way a person understands information. For example, if your friend is autistic they might concentrate on the exact meaning of words. Sometimes this can make sentences very confusing. For example, if you are waiting in a queue and a girl pushes to the front, you might say, 'That girl jumped in front of me!' Your autistic friend may think you mean the girl actually jumped up and down in front of you. Knowing how to respond to other people can be more difficult if you are autistic. However, being autistic can also help you think of interesting ideas that nobody else has thought of before!

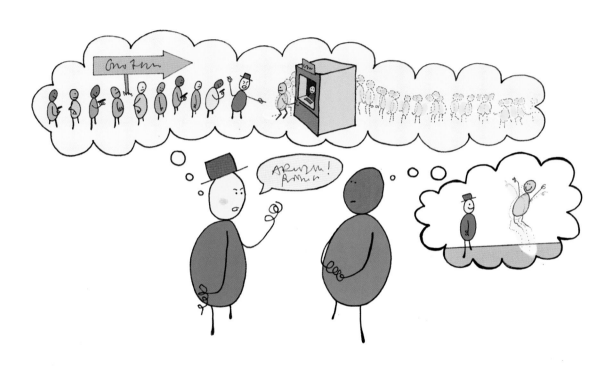

19. "Are there differences between autistic boys and autistic girls?"

Autistic girls are usually more interested in friendship groups and they can be very good at learning things by watching their friends. Autistic girls often find it easier to hide their worries. Sometimes autistic boys can find it harder to stay calm when they are feeling angry or upset. This could be why some doctors and teachers find it easier to notice when a boy is autistic.

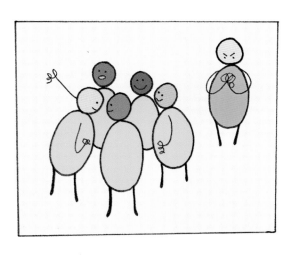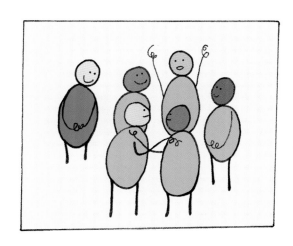

20. "My friend is autistic, will she be able to do the same things as me when she grows up?"

Everybody is different and we all have different abilities. Some autistic adults need help with everyday things such as eating and communicating. Other autistic adults go to university and learn to drive a car. Your friend will always have autism and there are some things she might do differently to you. Your friend might do the same amount of things as you or she might do even more than you. Remember, you don't have to do exactly the same things to be good friends!

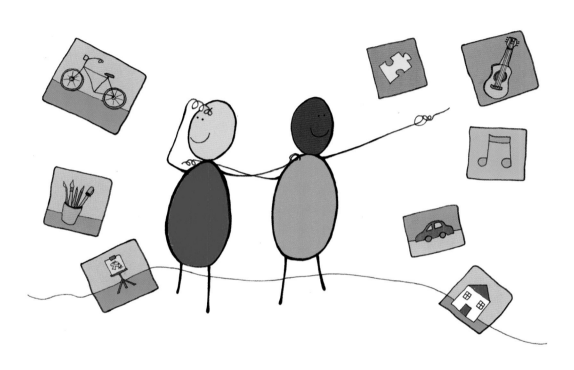

21. "How can I be a good friend to someone who is autistic?"

One of the best things you can do is learn about autism. The more you learn, the more considerate and understanding you can be. Everyone is different, so get to know your friend and see what they enjoy doing. Find out if there are any activities you can do together and invite them to join in. Autism changes the way a person understands the world, so your friend might have lots of interesting ideas to share with you!

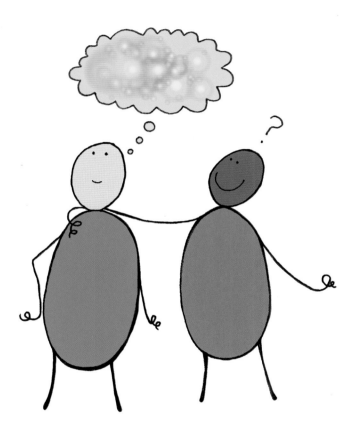

What Is It Like to Live with Autism?

Dear Parents, Schools, Teachers and Allies,

In this chapter we look at some of the questions students have asked in relation to living with autism. We invite readers to consider the reasons an autistic person might feel uncomfortable making eye contact and we explore the ways in which sensory input can affect individuals on the spectrum.

A Parent's Perspective...

One of the most valuable ways you can support readers to understand autism is to empower them with information they can relate to. Understanding the significance of sensory overload is far easier when you discuss an experience that makes the topic relatable. For example, recalling the intense sensation of a chilli pepper that feels too spicy or the sound of nails on a chalkboard. Once you have captured the

imagination of a young person, you can explain that everybody has different sensory thresholds. A sound that one person barely notices might be an unbearable distraction for a person with sensory sensitivity.

In this chapter we address a question about repetitive behaviours, often referred to as self-stimulation or 'stimming'. These behaviours are described by many autistic people as a vital means of 'self-regulation'. Stimming can be a self-soothing activity, an expression of anxiety, a form of pleasure or a method of processing sensory stimuli. It is often met with surprise and confusion, yet it is a behaviour exhibited by all of us, to some degree. We are all familiar with the impatient tapping of fingernails, the sound of optimistic humming or the flapping of hands around a person's mouth when they taste a curry that is too spicy for them. If an autistic individual is hypersensitive, they may find themselves overwhelmed by stimuli that others barely notice. We invite you to discuss sensory experiences and consider the fact that everybody processes sensory information differently. It makes no sense to judge a person's stimming based on your own sensory threshold. The world may feel neutral to you, but what if the world feels like a spicy curry to someone else? Hand flapping may be the most natural and appropriate response for them, regardless of how you feel. Autistic people can also experience hyposensitivity and may exhibit stimming behaviours because they are seeking sensory input.

We have attempted to distill complex information into bite-sized pieces that can be easily digested and discussed. We offer young readers information to help them understand the way autism might affect somebody's brain and we address questions about autism and learning.

While embracing the curiosity of young readers, try encouraging them to consider their motivation for asking questions. Support them to frame questions with respect and sensitivity and challenge them to reflect on different ways they can put their learning to good use.

In what ways can you use the information in this book to be more considerate and understanding of others?

22. "How do lights, noises and smells affect autistic people?"

Being autistic can make you extra sensitive. Everyday things like supermarket lights and busy places can feel very uncomfortable. Noises that don't bother anyone else might be painful and distracting for an autistic person. Sometimes all the sights, sounds, smells and feelings can get too difficult to cope with. If an autistic person can't cope, they might cry, panic or move about in a way you didn't expect. Sometimes you might see an autistic person wearing headphones to block out noises. Being autistic can also make you *less* sensitive to certain things. Some autistic people enjoy tight hugs, sparkly lights and making loud noises.

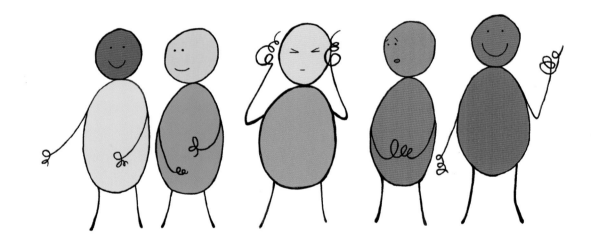

23. "My cousin is autistic, why does she find it difficult to look at me when we're talking?"

Eye contact can feel very uncomfortable for some autistic people. Your cousin might prefer to look away when you are talking, but that doesn't mean she isn't listening. Autism can make it difficult for your cousin to concentrate on looking at your face while listening to what you're saying at the same time. She might be looking away because she is concentrating on what you are saying.

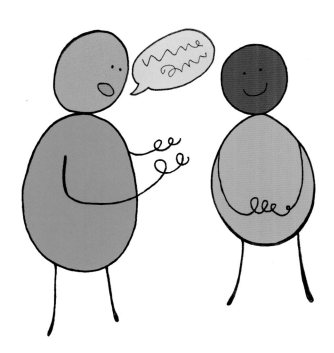

24. "Why does my autistic friend do things over and over again?"

Everybody fidgets, hums or taps their feet sometimes. We do this when we feel bored, anxious or excited. It's exactly the same for your friend but they might do it more often. An autistic person might bounce their legs or tap their fingers to help them stay calm when they are feeling worried or frustrated. It's exactly the same as when you eat something too spicy and you flap your hands around your mouth. Some autistic people repeat words to help them understand what is being said to them or because it feels good. If you are autistic you might wave your hands around when you are feeling happy or excited.

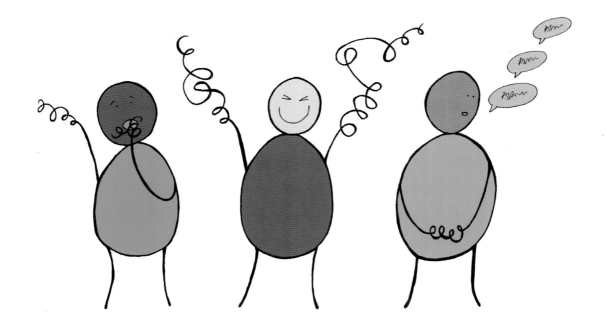

25. "Does autism run in families?"

Sometimes autism can run in families. This means autism can be common amongst members of the same family. Some scientists believe there may be 'autism genes' that cause autism. We all have thousands of genes inside our bodies that make us who we are. Your genes come from your birth family. If there are lots of people with brown eyes in your birth family, you might have brown eyes too. If you have autism, there might be other people in your family who have autism as well.

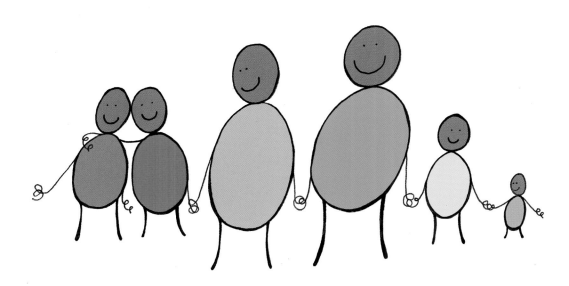

26. "What does autism do to your brain?"

Your brain is made up of different parts. Each part is in charge of a different job, like seeing, hearing, tasting and feeling. The different parts of your brain send signals to each other and this helps you to understand the world around you. Some scientists think that autism changes your brain signals. This means that autism changes the way your brain understands the world.

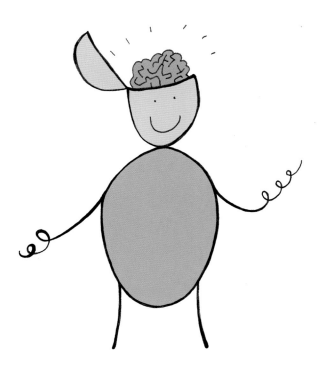

27. "Does autism affect learning at school?"

Sometimes autism affects learning at school because it affects the way you listen and communicate. Autism can make it more difficult to follow instructions and understand other people. However, autistic people can think very logically and some autistic people enjoy subjects like maths, science and IT because of the way their brain works. Being autistic can make you sensitive to noises that don't bother anyone else so you might find it harder to concentrate if people are talking during lessons. If you are autistic, you might need extra breaks at school and that's OK. With the right support everybody can take part in learning.

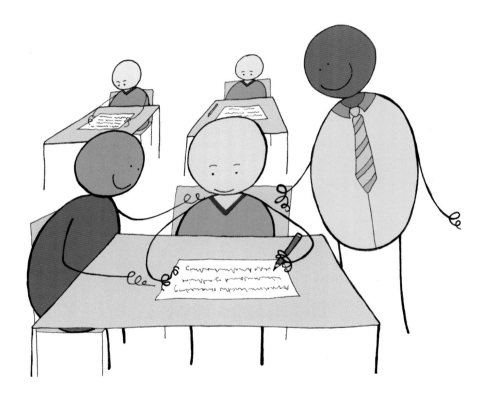

28. "Can you grow out of autism?"

Autism is something you are born with and you cannot grow out of it. If you are autistic, you will always be autistic. Some people like being autistic and they wouldn't want to grow out of it, even if they could. It's good to focus on your strengths and abilities. If you find something difficult you can practise and learn new skills. With the right support, some autistic children can turn their favourite hobbies into brilliant careers when they grow up.

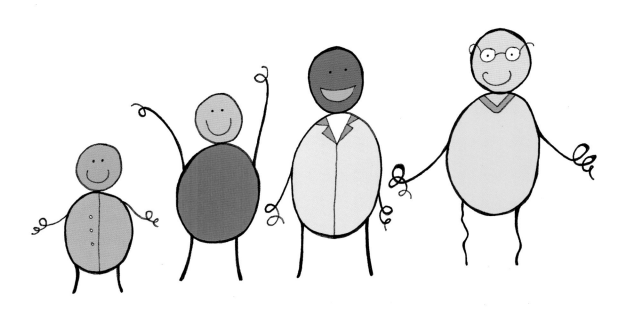

Is It OK for Me to Ask Questions?

Dear Parents, Schools, Teachers and Allies,

In this final chapter we will take a look at some of the more difficult and unusual questions students have asked us. We consider questions such as 'Can autism make you die?', 'Can you catch autism?' and 'Can pets have autism?' In collaboration with individuals from the autism community, we have created answers that act as a platform for meaningful discussion and further exploration, both at home and in the classroom. We invite you to consider how adults respond to questions about sensitive topics and what kind of message is being conveyed when we say, *'You mustn't ask that!'*

Young learners often ask very honest and direct questions. This can provide useful insight into their current understanding of autism and will highlight areas that need addressing. Try working with their natural curiosity and recognise when a conversation is being avoided because a question is deemed too difficult or controversial.

We encourage you to explore why certain questions might be problematic and to consider how they might be re-phrased. Focus on building a safe space where difficult issues can be explored with sensitivity and respect. In the classroom, some autistic students will discuss their autism with enthusiasm and other students may not wish to share their experiences at all. Acknowledge and accommodate the unique preferences of your students and support their peers to do the same.

A Parent's Perspective...

We believe that it's OK to ask questions if you don't understand something. As one mother told us, 'You should just give people a chance to show themselves... When you say "I want to keep it secret", it's a bit like saying there's something to be ashamed of. There's nothing to be ashamed of.'

29. "Is autism a disability?"

Disability means different things to different people. Some people call autism a disability because it can make life very challenging. Other people call autism a 'difference' because it gives them a different way of thinking. Many autistic people are proud of their differences. It's important to celebrate autistic strengths.

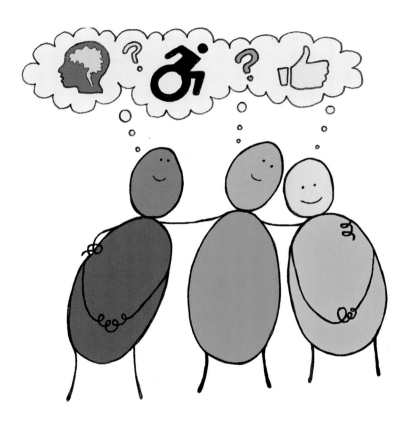

30. "How do you know if someone is autistic if you can't tell just by looking at them?"

Autism is sometimes called an 'invisible' condition, because it's hard to see if a person is autistic just by looking at them. Autism doesn't affect the way you look. Autism affects a person's experiences, thoughts and behaviour. Doctors can tell if someone is autistic by spending time with them and asking them questions.

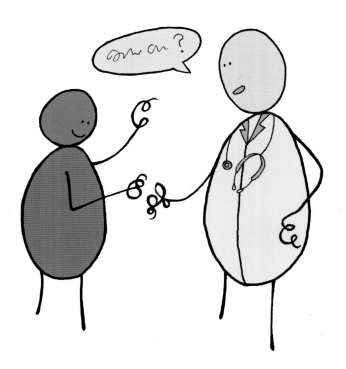

31. "Can pets be autistic?"

Autism is a condition that affects a person's brain. Most animals have brains too. We don't know if pets can be autistic yet. In the future, scientists might study intelligent animals like chimpanzees and dolphins to find out.

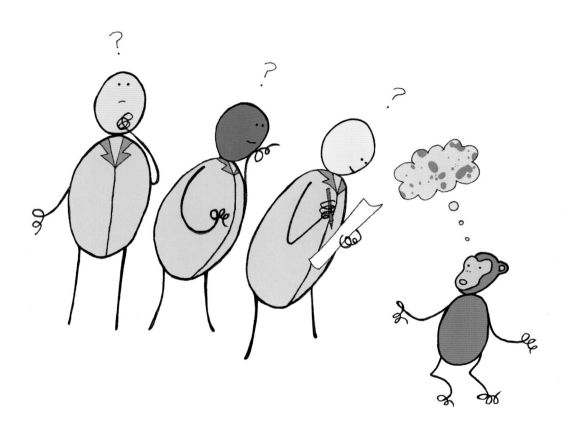

32. "Is it OK when someone is autistic?"

Yes, it's completely OK when someone is autistic. Autism can create challenges but that's OK. If you are autistic, you might need extra help at home, school or work. It's helpful if the people around you learn about autism. It's not OK if someone is left out because they are autistic. Many people are proud of their autism because it helps them to see the world in a unique way.

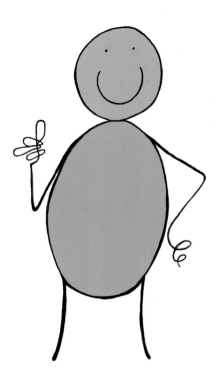

33. "Can you catch autism?"

No, autism is not a disease and it's not contagious.
You can't catch autism like you can catch a cold.
Autism has nothing to do with germs and it does not
spread. Even if all your friends were autistic, you still
wouldn't be able to catch it. Autism is something
that you are born with, like the colour of your hair.

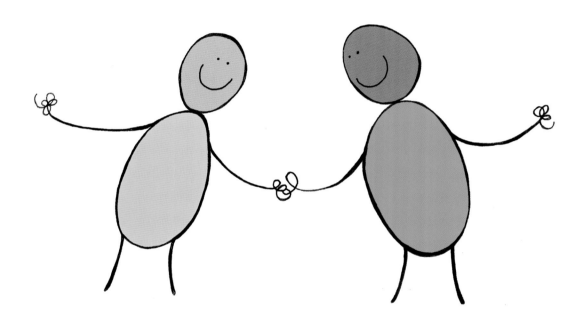

34. "Can you die from autism?"

No, autism is not an illness. If you are autistic you can still get sick like everybody else, but you can't die from autism. With good health and the right support, all of us can live long and happy lives.

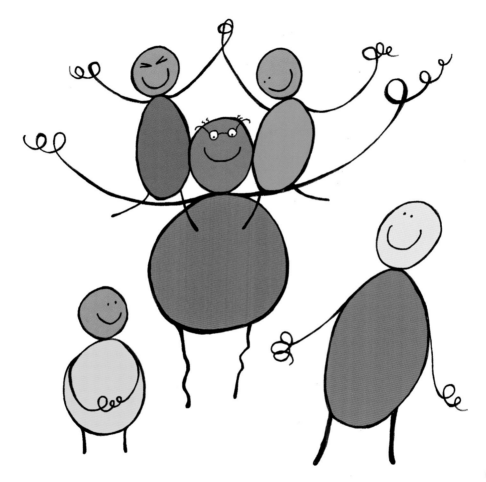

35. "Is it normal for people to feel uncomfortable around autistic people?"

Lots of us feel uncomfortable around behaviour we don't understand. However, it's never OK to be unkind to someone just because you don't understand them. Remember, the world can be very confusing and uncomfortable for autistic people too. Learning about autism will help you to be more comfortable and more considerate.

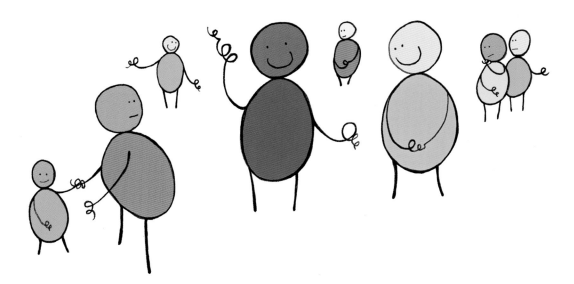

Ten Tips for Teachers

1. **Each student with autism is different:** What works well for one student won't necessarily work for another. A behaviour trigger for one student might not even faze another student.

2. **Give clear and direct instructions:** Students with autism can be very literal thinkers. Avoid statements such as, 'You have left such a mess by the sink!' To a student with autism, you may simply be making an observation or stating a fact. Instead use clear and direct language such as, 'Go and clean your paintbrush and put your paper towel in the bin.'

3. **Modify class work and the classroom environment:** Many students with autism have difficulty with executive-functioning skills. This can impact on their ability to listen, focus, complete tasks and be organised. A distraction-free desk and a lesson broken down into small chunks, with 'brain breaks' will work wonders for students with autism.

4. **Encourage and re-direct:** Focus on promoting and encouraging positive behaviour with rewards and praise. Re-direct inappropriate behaviour and notice how you respond to the behaviour. If a student seeks your attention by shouting out when you have already asked them to raise their hand, avoid engaging with the student until they have raised their hand. It may sound simple but it's very easy to encourage inappropriate behaviour without realising it.

5. **Social stress:** Think about pairing a student with a playtime buddy or allowing them to access a lunchtime club to alleviate social isolation and anxiety at playtime. Support their peers to understand and respect neurodiversity. A person with autism may not be able to read vital social cues. They made need additional explanations for things that their peers understand

instinctively, for example how other people are feeling, non-verbal cues, facial expressions, intonation, body language and unspoken social rules.

6. **Focus on the positives:** Recognise and make the most of a student's talents and interests – if they like trains then it might be worth finding a train-related fractions worksheet or reward chart.

7. **Be alert for sensory needs:** A noisy cafeteria or bright lights in the assembly hall might be unbearable for a student with autism, so allow them to eat lunch elsewhere or skip assembly time. A lot of resistant behaviours come from sensory discomfort. Your student may not be able to tell you they are experiencing sensory issues. Educate yourself about sensory overload and 'stimming' behaviours.

8. **Help with transition times:** Classroom alterations and last-minute changes to the timetable could prove very difficult for a student with autism. Consider using a visual timetable and always talk about changes in advance, to reduce anxiety and outbursts of distress.

9. **Pick your moments:** Avoid disciplining a student when they are angry, over-stimulated, aggressive or emotional, as they will be unable to interact with you and comply with the consequence. Allow for time to calm down and then discuss their behaviour calmly and constructively.

10. **Learn about it:** Educate others about autism and talk about autism with the whole class, emphasising the individuality of each student and the positive aspects of autism.

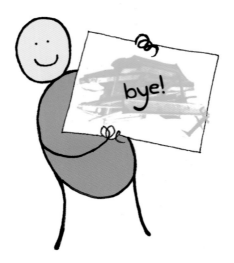